KENNEDY
SALAMAN

# PREVENTING AND CONQUERING Diabetes

Revolutionary Keys to Winning the Blood-Sugar Battle

STRATFORD
PUBLISHING

IMPORTANT NOTICE

This book is neither a medical guide nor a manual for self-treatment. It is instead intended as a reference work only. The information in this book is meant to help you make informed choices about your health, but is not intended as a substitute for any treatment that may be prescribed or recommended by your doctor or health care practitioner. If you should suspect that you suffer from a medical condition or problem, you should seek competent medical care without delay

*Diana Dalton has been an angel in my life who has lifted my feet when my wings have been too weak to fly. Because of her sustaining character, she will be my friend in this world and the next.*

***Preventing and Conquering Diabetes***



ISBN 0-913087-29-7

First Printing

MKS, Inc.
1259 El Camino Real, Suite 1500
Menlo Park, California 94025
www.mksalaman.com
(650) 854-3922 telephone
(650) 854-5779 facsimile

Distributed by:
Maximum Living, Inc.
20071 Soulsbyville Road
Soulsbyville, California 95372-9748
www.maximizeyourlife.com
(209) 536-9300 telephone
(800) 445-4325 toll-free
(209) 536-9375 facsimile

*Literary development and interior and cover design by:*
Koechel Peterson & Associates, Inc., Minneapolis, MN

Cover photo by Russ Fischella

Printed in the United States of America

# CONTENTS

CHAPTER ONE

# UNDERSTANDING DIABETES

*There are no such things as incurables; there are only things for which man has not found a cure.*

*—Bernard M. Baruch*

**HER FACE WAS AS WHITE AS A SHEET** when she fell against the wall, then slumped to the floor, quivering and shaking. "Quick, my purse," she finally choked, her voice barely a whisper.

I ran back to the nurse's station, feeling rather faint myself, fearing the worst. "Please, the nurse...she needs her purse," I blurted out to the woman behind the desk.

"Oh, Nancy!" the woman exclaimed. Moving with lightning speed, she grabbed a brown bag from under the counter and dashed into the hallway, reaching into Nancy's purse to retrieve her insulin.

Half an hour later, Nancy was recovering in the nurse's lounge, sipping a glass of orange juice. Her supervisor—the woman who came to her rescue—was explaining that Nancy gets so busy with her nursing duties she forgets to take her insulin and goes into shock. Fortunately, it doesn't happen often, and, also fortunately, Nancy works in a hospital and is around people who know what to do when time and self-awareness get away from her. Not every diabetic is so fortunate.

## THE REASONS FOR DIABETES

Diabetes occurs when the pancreas does not produce enough of the hormone insulin, which converts sugar, starches, and other food into energy and controls the level of blood sugar (glucose).

Nancy has Type 1 diabetes. It is usually diagnosed in children and young adults and was previously called insulin-dependent diabetes mellitus (IDDM) or juvenile-onset diabetes.

Similar to rheumatoid arthritis, lupus, and vitiligo, Type 1 diabetes is an autoimmune disease. It develops when the body's immune system destroys pancreatic beta cells, the only cells in the body that make insulin.

Insulin moves sugar from the blood into the cells. One of the first symptoms of diabetes is severe fatigue, as no sugar in the cells means no energy to the body. Another symptom is high blood sugar—hyperglycemia.

There is nothing so heartbreaking than the sight of a little child injecting himself with a hypodermic needle. For diabetics, the needle is their lifeline. In order to survive, people with Type 1 diabetes must have insulin delivered by a pump or injections. But insulin dependency is like turning off the smoke alarm without removing the cigarette left burning in the sofa.

The problem with depending on insulin instead of nutrition to control diabetes is that it doesn't deal with the resultant metabolic problems that occur. Arteriosclerosis (inflammation of the walls of the arteries) proceeds at five times the rate it does in the non-diabetic, causing a particular kind of heart disease, and circulatory problems that can lead to the loss of limbs, blindness, kidney failure, and early death.

Prescribed insulin does not cure the problem. It only alleviates the symptoms. Careful eating and knowledgeable supplementation can help reduce the need for insulin in Type 1s.

Type 2 diabetes is the most common form. In Type 2, either the body does not produce enough insulin or the cells ignore the insulin. Ninety percent of those with diabetes have Type 2, and it is estimated that 90 percent of them are obese. Sometimes called "adult onset diabetes," it is typically diagnosed among middle-aged, overweight, inactive people. Unfortunately, more and more people with Type 2 are children.

Less than two decades ago, Type 2 diabetes was virtually unheard of among children and accounted for less than 3 percent of new diabetes cases among children and adolescents. But a new study shows that Type 2 diabetes now accounts for up to 45 percent of new diabetes cases among adolescents worldwide. The rate of Type 2 diabetes among younger children is also rising dramatically.

What we also know, now, is that dietary changes, nutritional supplementation, weight loss, and exercise can reverse the diabetic condition among Type 2s.

## THE ROLE OF SUGAR

It is easy to be confused about blood sugar when it comes to diabetes. If a lack of sugar is the problem, you might think eating sugar is the solution. However, eating more sugar does not put it in the cells where it is needed, only in the blood where the high amounts become toxic and cause complications, such as arteriosclerosis and kidney disease.

Whether it is Type 1 or Type 2, eating simple carbohydrates, such as refined sugar, only make the problem worse. The addition of refined sugar to most processed food and the increase in consumption of convenience foods are the likely reasons why diabetes has increased over the decades.

Refined sugar exhausts the pancreas, which is charged with producing insulin. The definitive essay on the subject is Surgeon-Captain T. L. Cleave's book, *The Saccharine Disease* (Keats Publishing Inc., 1975). Cleave shows example after example of societies in which the addition of sugar to the diet was the obvious starting point for the development of diabetes and of atherosclerosis in the epidemic proportions typical of a Western nation.

Two striking examples in Cleave's global studies were in Iceland beginning in 1920 and among the nomadic Yemenite Jews. Before sugar was introduced in their cultures, there was absolutely no diabetes or atherosclerosis. Two decades after their diets became similar to ours, because sugar was added, they began to develop nearly as high an incidence of these illnesses as we have.

Another of Cleave's great contributions was the discovery of the Law of Twenty Years. In every culture he studied, it took exactly twenty years after their dietary change for the first cases of diabetes and atherosclerosis to appear. In American terms, this means that the increase in consumption of sugar and highly refined flour between 1895 and 1910 can easily explain the beginning of the era of the heart attack and the increase in diabetes noted between 1910 and 1930. This increase has continued. In the years between 1935 and 1968, the prevalence has increased by 600 percent.

In the United States, inappropriate diet, such as the processed sugar already mentioned, is probably the major factor associated with insulin sensitivity and thus the major cause of diabetes.

## MINIMIZING THE RISK—MANAGING YOUR DIABETES

You've finished the first step: understanding diabetes and why it occurs. Now for the second step: how to use the principles of diabetes to both monitor and control your diabetic condition and prevent complications from occurring.

CHAPTER TWO

# GLYCEMIC INDEX FOODS THAT CONTROL BLOOD SUGAR

*Give us this day our daily bread (but, please, none of the white processed kind).*

**BEFORE I BEGIN, PLEASE CONSIDER** the following important facts about white bread, which I like to call "glue food."

- More than 98 percent of convicted felons are bread users.
- Fully HALF of all children who grow up in bread-consuming households score below average on standardized tests.
- More than 90 percent of violent crimes are committed within 24 hours of eating bread.
- Primitive tribal societies that eat no commercial bread exhibit a low incidence of diabetes, cancer, Alzheimer's, Parkinson's disease, and osteoporosis.

- Bread has been proven to be addictive. Subjects deprived of bread and given only water begged for bread after as little as two days.

In light of these and other frightening statistics, we propose the following bread restrictions:

- No sale of bread to minors.
- A nationwide "Just Say No to Toast" campaign, complete with celebrity TV spots and bumper stickers.
- A 300 percent federal tax on all bread to pay for weight-loss programs.
- No animal or human images or any primary colors (which may appeal to children) may be used to promote bread usage.
- The establishment of "Bread-free" zones around schools.

Okay, some of this is tongue-in-cheek, but in this chapter you'll see that bread and other foods like it are the dietary root of diabetic evils.

## A NEW STRATEGY FOR CONTROLLING BLOOD SUGAR

Eliminating refined bread, such as the common "white" bread, and foods like it are the first steps toward controlling blood sugar levels, and thus the damaging effects of diabetes. The best time to determine your blood sugar level is after you eat.

Over the course of a day, it's normal for your blood sugar level to go up and down. The specific amount of sugar in the blood at any given time is known as your "free blood glucose level."

Before a meal, free blood glucose levels are generally low. After a meal, the free blood glucose level rises as food is digested, and then gradually returns to a lower level as insulin is released from the pancreas and the body's cells take glucose from the blood and use it for energy. In diabetics, blood sugar levels stay as high as the food raised them.

This is why what you eat is so important to control blood sugar. Eat the wrong foods, and your blood sugar level will go out of control. When this happens often enough, serious problems occur.

People with Type 1 diabetes can reduce the risk of the complications—including the ones leading to blindness, kidney failure, and amputation—by as much as 76 percent by keeping blood sugar to normal or near-normal levels. Other studies have shown reductions in complications of up to 70 percent for Type 2 patients.

What if the food eaten did not raise blood sugar to critical levels? Not all carbohydrates are created equal, nor will they all affect your blood sugar in the same way. Researchers have created a Glycemic Index that ranks foods according to their ability to raise blood sugar. Where do you think bread ranks?

## WHAT IS THE GLYCEMIC INDEX?

The speed at which a food is able to increase a person's blood glucose levels is called the *glycemic response.* The glycemic response is influenced by many factors. Some factors may be the amount of food you eat (ideally small portions), how the food is processed (as little as possible), or the way the food is prepared. For instance, pasta cooked *al dente* (firm) is absorbed more slowly than pasta that is overcooked.

Essentially, the Glycemic Index is based on how quickly a particular food is digested, metabolized, and then released into the bloodstream as sugar/glucose. It is a ranking of foods based on their immediate effects on blood sugar levels and measures how much a person's blood glucose increases over a period of two or three hours after a meal. A food with a moderate Glycemic Index can be lowered by cooking or processing it less and made even lower by eating small portions slowly. You will find a list of foods and their rankings at the end of this chapter.

Using home glucose tests, diabetics can create their own Glycemic Index by testing blood sugar before and after meals, then recording the results. This is a good idea since each individual might have a different response to specific foods due to food sensitivities or food allergies.

The index ranks food on a scale of 0 to 100, indicating whether a food will raise blood glucose just a little, moderately, or dramatically. The lower the number, the slower the action and the better for diabetics. The higher the number, the quicker the rise in blood sugar—not good for diabetics.

Foods with a low number, by the way, also burn fat, helping the diabetic lose weight, which is another way to control the diabetic condition. More on that later.

## GI FOOD VALUES

Now that I've sold you on the concept, here is what you've been waiting for: the carbohydrate foods with low Glycemic Index rankings. As a general rule, anything *processed* for fast digestion will have a high Glycemic Index (GI). Hence, fast food usually has a high GI.

A GI of 70 or more is high, a GI of 56 to 69 is medium, and a GI of 55 or less is low.

Where do you think bread ranks? The highest GI food is commonly found on the American dinner plate: white bread. It's in pizza and most every fast food meal out there. The rank of white bread is 100.

Pasta has a low Glycemic Index. Why? Because it is prepared from semolina or cracked wheat, not wheat flour. The method of preparation is important, because the large particle size means that we absorb it more slowly. In general, when you choose pasta, spend a little more to get a better product.

On a personal note, I have made several changes in my diet on the basis of what I've learned about the Glycemic Index. One change I made was to eat barley, because barley has such a low index, about 46, and it is high in chromium and fiber, about which I will also explain later.

Another change was that I eat a lot of chana dal, otherwise known as Bengal gram dal (cicer arietinum). This is a split yellow legume, similar to garbanzo beans (chick peas) but smaller and sweeter. Clinical trials from India and South Africa show a Glycemic Index of 11 and 7 respectively, just about the lowest Glycemic Index of any food tested. This food, generally available in East Indian food stores, not only has a remarkably low index, but it also has a wonderful flavor.

Foods such as milk and fruit have a lower Glycemic Index value than common starchy foods, such as bread, rice, potatoes, and breakfast cereals.

The good news is foods that were previously avoided by people with diabetes can now be added to their diet in moderation, since we know it's not how much sugar is in the food, it's how fast the food releases sugar into the bloodstream.

Most low glycemic foods are high in fiber and low in fat. This includes fruit, legumes, barley, pasta, and whole grains (e.g., cracked wheat).

Here are some tips for low glycemic, diabetic-friendly meals:

- Prepare dishes with beans, such as chili, soups, and salad.
- Eat whole grain, pumpernickel, and oat bran bread.
- Eat fresh fruit.
- Eat parboiled, brown, or whole grain rice instead of instant rice.

- Eat pasta, rice, yams, lima beans, or baked potatoes instead of mashed, boiled, or instant potatoes.
- For between meal snacks, eat nuts. Almonds are not only 0 on the Glycemic Index, but the oleic acid they contain enhances beta cell efficiency. One study of Type 2 diabetics found that 70 percent were able to reduce their medications while maintaining an almond-rich diet.

**LOW TO MEDIUM GLYCEMIC INDEX FOODS**

| | |
|---|---|
| Popcorn | 58 |
| Oat bran bread | 68 |
| Oatmeal (slow cook oats) | 70 |
| Parboiled rice | 68 |
| Pumpernickel | 66 |
| All-Bran | 60 |
| Sweet potato | 54 |
| Skim milk | 46 |
| Pasta | 40 to 70 |
| Lentils/kidney/baked beans | 40 to 69 |
| Apple/banana/plum | 34 to 69 |
| Nuts | 0 to 10 |

**AVOID THESE HIGH GLYCEMIC INDEX FOODS**

| | |
|---|---|
| Instant rice | 124 |
| Corn flake cereal | 119 |
| Crisped rice cereal | 117 |
| Jellybeans | 114 |

| | |
|---|---|
| French fries | 107 |
| Soda crackers | 106 |
| Potato (boiled or mashed) | 104 |
| White bread | 100 |
| Melba toast | 100 |
| Couscous | 93 |
| Ice cream | 87 |
| Oatmeal (quick cook) | 87 |
| Table sugar (sucrose) | 83 |

It would be impossible to list every food and its index rating. If you have access to the Internet and want to know the rating of a specific food such as an apple, search for "glycemic apple." This technique is widely used, and there is much information available.

**TAKE CONTROL OF YOUR DIET**

The most important thing to remember about diabetes is that you are not helpless. You are not a slave to your hypodermic needle or to your doctor. With the help of this booklet, you can take control of your diet and make a difference in it.

CHAPTER THREE

# GETTING DOWN TO BASICS

*To eat is human; to digest, divine.*

*—C. T. Copeland*

**YOU KNOW YOU NEED TO** do something about your weight when you board an airplane and the flight attendant designates your stomach as carry-on luggage. Notorious Heide has it so bad she needs control top turtlenecks.

In the Academy Award winning film documentary *Super Size Me,* Morgan Spurlock goes on a quest to answer the question, "Why are Americans so fat?" His pursuit led him to examine the effects of a steady diet of fast food by eating three meals every day at McDonald's for one month. During those 30 days, his cholesterol jumped 65 points, he gained 24.5 pounds, his blood pressure skyrocketed, and he suffered from depression and rapid mood swings. They were afraid it was going to kill him.

## THE ROOT OF DIABETIC EVIL

I am convinced that today's modern diet of denatured, processed, and chemicalized food, which includes white bread ("glue food"), is the root of diabetic evil.

Whole civilizations previously exempt, once introduced to affluence and its accompanying Western diet high in fat and sugar, have found themselves in an epidemic of diabetes.

What is it about our modern-day diet that contributes to diabetes? Fat, sugar, and inactivity. Poor circulation from a lack of exercise causes a lack of oxygen to the cells and allows a poor diet to affect the health. Our modern diet is full of unhealthy trans-fatty and saturated fats. Fat in the bloodstream blocks the effectiveness of insulin and increases the chances that diabetes will lead to more severe problems. Chemical preservatives, colorings, and emulsifiers alter the body's natural workings extensively and can contribute to blood sugar issues.

Fortunately, there is much that can be done to overcome poor eating habits, even decades' worth.

## EXERCISE AFTER YOU EAT

Studies also show that exercise affects those with diabetes differently than those without it. When people with healthy insulin activity exercise, their blood sugar levels rise. But when diabetics exercise, their blood sugar levels do not rise, demonstrating that exercise is particularly beneficial for those with both Type 1 and Type 2 diabetes, even without the weight-loss benefit.

Every diabetic, regardless of age or type, should be in a fitness protection program. Exercise not only loses the fat but lowers blood sugar and improves the health of body cells, making them insulin sensitive. The cells of "exercising" muscles can extract glucose from the blood much more effectively than resting muscles.

The best part? The exercise need not be strenuous or lengthy. Researchers have found that moderate exercise has a more profound effect on blood sugar levels among those with diabetes than in normal individuals.

## FIBER LOWERS INSULIN NEEDS

A high fiber diet helps both obese and lean diabetics, according to researchers. Both groups reduced blood fats and the need for insulin through a high fiber diet.

Fiber is one of the best dietary aids for weight loss and blood sugar control, because it moves food quickly through the digestive system, slows down the absorption of simple carbohydrates, and minimizes the release of glucose, decreasing the Glycemic Index of other foods eaten.

With fiber, most think of bran wheat, rye, oat, or rice. But the range of fibers goes beyond grains to beans, lentils, vegetables, and fruit. While wheat bran rates highest in fiber content, blackberries, dried prunes, and apples with skin are excellent. Vegetables such as celery and carrots rate high, too.

Since the average American diet contains between 11 and 21 grams of fiber daily, diabetics need to double or triple their fiber intake. I suggest doing this by eating one high fiber food a day, particularly whole grains and beans, and increasing fluid intake to help the body adjust to increased gas, a common side effect of added fiber.

Outstanding fiber foods are almonds, apples, blackberries, broccoli, corn, fresh peas, kidney beans, plums, potatoes, prunes, raisins, spinach, sweet potatoes, whole wheat bread, figs, and zucchini. Outstanding fiber supplements (food derived in a formula) are psyllium, hyssop, oat bran, alfalfa, rhubarb, and buckthorn.

Psyllium and hyssop are two excellent sources of dietary fiber. Psyllium, known for its cholesterol-lowering properties, and hyssop, valued as an excellent source of fiber, is contained in Maximum Living's Hyssop Cleanse, which contains all the best sources of fiber, not just the main two.

David, of the Bible, knew the benefits of hyssop. He drew lessons from the remedy, which he used in showing the cleansing of the body from sin, for he said, "Purge me with hyssop, and I shall be clean; wash me, and I shall be whiter than snow" (Psalms 51:7).

## GLUCOSE-REGULATING FOODS

Before you examine foods that control blood sugar levels, consider the possibility they may be *causing* it. Diabetics should be thoroughly tested for food allergies that may contribute to the disease by causing inflammation and autoimmune destruction of the insulin-producing cells of the pancreas. Foods that often are associated with diabetes-related problems include corn, wheat, chocolate, and dairy products.

The Glycemic Index is one way to choose foods for the diabetic diet. But there are foods close to nature—God-given foods, back-to-basic foods—that have such reputations for helping the diabetic condition that they should be mentioned.

Broiled stems of the Mexican opuntia cactus—the genus Opuntia Streptacantha Lemaire—help to control non-insulin dependent diabetes by lowering blood glucose and insulin levels, say Mexican scientists. This cactus, whose broiled stems serve as a common food in arid parts of Mexico, can also be found in the deserts of the southwestern United States. Ask for the plant at your health food store. Sometimes a dried version is available.

Aloe vera juice, a traditional diabetic remedy in Arabia, has been found to lower blood sugar in diabetics. Researchers at Fujita Health University in Japan found when aloe was given to diabetics, their fasting blood glucose level went down.

Through the years in folk medicine, legumes—beans, peas, and lentils—have led the pack for controlling blood sugar. Beans are rich in soluble fibers that lower blood cholesterol and blood sugar. One-half to one cup of beans per day can significantly reduce blood cholesterol levels and help control blood sugar levels of people who have Type 2 diabetes.

While studying soybeans' ability to lower cholesterol, biochemist scientists discovered that soybeans also keep insulin levels under control. Soybeans are high in fiber, flavonoids, and protein and are low on the Glycemic Index.

People with high blood sugar should eat at least two meals a day of legumes. Good ideas are lentil stew or soup for breakfast and pinto beans for dinner. Lentils are complex carbohydrates, excellent for controlling blood sugar and encouraging an energetic start to the day. And if weight is a problem, lentils can help control the appetite as well. To remove some of the troublesome carbohydrates, soak dry beans in water for three to five hours and discard this water before cooking. To retain all the nutrients, use this water and eat alone.

The flavonoid rutin is one of the reasons for buckwheat's blood sugar lowering properties. The common belief is that buckwheat is a cereal grain, but it is actually a fruit seed that is related to rhubarb and sorrel. In a placebo-controlled study, a single dose of buckwheat seed extract lowered blood glucose levels by 12 to 19 percent at 90 and 120 minutes after being fed to rats with chemically-induced diabetes.

If you use buckwheat in your recipes, use the whole seed, not flour. The best way to avoid the hazards of processed flour is to grind the seed yourself and make your own flour, thus retaining the nutrients.

## THE SPICES OF LIFE

Certain spices have been found to lower blood sugar. The newest discovery is cinnamon, which was found to increase the metabolism of glucose by 20 times. It didn't matter what form or type of cinnamon it was—all worked. One scientist recommended that diabetics take a half to 1 teaspoon ground cinnamon daily. I'll take mine in applesauce, thank you.

Fenugreek seeds are a good source of soluble fiber, and in animal experiments the spice has been found to lower blood sugar and cholesterol as well. Researchers in India found that glucose tolerance improved, urinary glucose excretion decreased 70 percent, and insulin responses were reduced in people with diabetes after defatted fenugreek was used for 10 days.

Fenugreek is a favorite in northern African and Middle Eastern dishes and is one of the few spices that is usually used in powdered form even in Indian curries. Seed extract is used in breads in Egypt and Ethiopia. Ground seeds can give a nice lift to some bland vegetarian dishes and are also good in marinades.

Linseed also provides benefits to people with diabetes. Subjects consuming bread containing 25 percent linseed meal showed an almost 30 percent improvement in a glucose tolerance test. Linseed is a close cousin to flaxseed, which is beneficial as a supplement. More on this later.

Traditional herbalism places great value on European blueberry leaves, a.k.a. bilberry, as a natural method of controlling or lowering blood sugar levels when they are slightly elevated. Results have shown the leaves have an active ingredient with a remarkable ability to reduce excess sugar in the blood. More on bilberry later, in relation to diabetic retinopathy.

Other spices/herbs found to benefit the diabetic condition are garlic, onions, bay leaves, cloves, cumin, and turmeric.

## FINE TUNE YOUR CONTROL

What is in food that controls blood sugar? In the next chapter, I will show you how to multiply the glucose-control benefit of food by targeting supplements that contain their active ingredients.

CHAPTER FOUR

# SUPPLEMENTAL SAFEGUARDS

*Joy and Temperance and*
*Repose slam the door*
*on the doctor's nose.*

*—Henry Wadsworth Longfellow*

**THE YEAR WAS 1968,** and a little boy accompanied his mother to the river to pick blackberries. Engrossed in filling his pail while trying to avoid the scratchy thorns, he failed to notice his mother kneeling on the ground. The sound of her first heavy sob broke his concentration, and he dropped the pail, running to her. "What's wrong, Mama?" he implored. "What's wrong?"

Billy's mama had just learned that his six-year-old sister, Margie, had juvenile diabetes, and that Margie would be lucky if she lived to see her thirty-second birthday. This tragic reality, according to a life insurance study, was the average life expectancy for children under the age of 15 diagnosed with juvenile diabetes from 1950 to 1971.

Before the health food and supplement industry became mainstream, people were dependent on conventional medicine, and their prospects were heartbreaking.

Today a diagnosis of diabetes is still heart-wrenching. Since it is a metabolic dysfunction, it will change your life. No longer can you take good health for granted. Suddenly it is crucial that you know exactly how your body is functioning and what it needs to maintain health and vitality.

One of the first courses of action is to get a complete nutrition blood analysis, to determine if deficiencies could be making the condition worse. This is important because studies show many people with diabetes are nutritionally deficient, and this could contribute, or even cause, the problem.

An article in the *American Journal of Clinical Nutrition* reviewed 247 studies regarding the nutritional status of diabetics. It was found that Type 1 diabetics had deficiencies in the minerals zinc, calcium, magnesium, and vitamin D. Those with Type 2 diabetes were found to be low in the minerals zinc, magnesium, and vitamins B6 and C.

Deficiencies are important, but they are not the only story. Deficiencies revealed by tests only show what is missing to maintain health, not what is needed to overcome the diabetic condition. There are supplemental nutrients that effectively normalize blood sugar and help prevent the horrible side effects experienced by many diabetics.

## MINERAL SUPPLEMENTS

The first category of supplements is minerals. The diabetic condition itself may be the cause of mineral deficiencies. Elevated blood sugars stimulate excessive urination, which can wash essential minerals and trace elements out of the body.

Many diabetics are taking hypertensive medication and/or diuretics. Diuretics are notorious eliminators of all minerals, yet potassium is the only mineral routinely replaced.

### *Chromium*

Certain nutrients are essential for normal blood sugar levels and insulin absorption. Among these, the mineral chromium gets star billing. Thirty-five years of research on this mega-mineral suggest a deficiency of chromium increases the risk of developing diabetes.

Double-blind research shows that chromium supplements improve glucose tolerance in people with both Type 1 and Type 2 diabetes by increasing sensitivity to insulin. Chromium improves the processing of glucose in people with pre-diabetic glucose intolerance and in women with diabetes associated with pregnancy (gestational diabetes).

Dr. Walter Mertz has been documenting the effect of chromium on diabetes since the late 1920s and to this day advocates its use. He has shown conclusively that chromium is a crucial part of a substance termed the Glucose Tolerance

Factor (GTF), which includes chromium. When enough chromium is present in the diet, intestinal bacteria can manufacture GTF in the body.

Brewer's yeast is a good source of GTF. Both brewer's yeast (9 gm/day) and chromium (150 to 1,000 mcg/day) improves blood sugar metabolism when taken for several weeks to months. As a side benefit, brewer's yeast and chromium help lower bad cholesterol (LDL) and raise good cholesterol (HDL).

Brewer's yeast contains a particularly well-absorbed form of chromium, as does cheese, wheat germ, and organic, range-fed liver. Chromium is also found in whole grains, potatoes, and apples with skin, spinach, oysters, carrots, and chicken breast. Barley grown in Mesopotamia is said to be a rich source of chromium.

Some diabetics who required insulin shots to maintain their blood sugar at safe levels were able to get by on lower doses after taking chromium. It is estimated that probably one-fourth to one-half of the people in the United States are deficient in chromium.

### *Vanadium—Vanadyl Sulfate*

Another exceptionally useful trace mineral to combat diabetes is vanadium, which lowers blood sugar by mimicking insulin and improving the cells' sensitivity to insulin. A growing body of human research shows that vanadium compounds, most notably vanadyl sulfate, consistently improve fasting glucose and other measures of diabetes. These benefits were often extended for weeks after the mineral supplementation was discontinued.

Vanadium is a compound found in tiny amounts in plants and animals. Early studies showed that vanadium normalized blood glucose levels in animals with Type 1 and Type 2 diabetes. An Italian study found that vanadium has insulin-like effects on glucose metabolism. In animal studies, insulin-deficient rats showed markedly decreased blood glucose levels when given vanadium. In healthy individuals, from 100 to 300 micrograms a day is recommended. Foods lavish in vanadium are vegetable oils, whole grains, seafood, and organic, range-fed liver.

### *Manganese*

Manganese is an important cofactor in the key enzymes of glucose metabolism. A deficiency of manganese was found to result in diabetes in guinea pigs. It also resulted in the frequent birth of offspring that develop pancreatic abnormalities or no pancreas at all. Diabetics have been shown to have only one-half the manganese of normal individuals.

### *Potassium*

Insulin shots often cause a potassium deficiency, so supplementing with potassium is essential. This mineral also improves insulin sensitivity.

*Zinc*

A zinc deficiency may play a role in the development of diabetes. Zinc is involved in virtually all aspects of insulin metabolism—synthesis, secretion, and utilization. Zinc also has a protective effect against beta cell destruction and has well-known antiviral effects.

Zinc supplements have lowered blood sugar levels in people with Type 1. People with Type 2 diabetes also have low zinc levels, caused by excess loss of zinc in their urine.

*Magnesium*

Magnesium levels are significantly lowered in diabetics, and lowest in those with severe retinopathy. Studies suggest that a deficiency in magnesium may worsen the blood sugar control in Type 2 diabetes. A deficiency of magnesium interrupts insulin secretion in the pancreas and increases insulin resistance in the body's tissues.

Supplementation with magnesium leads to improved insulin production in elderly people with Type 2 diabetes. Elders without diabetes may also produce more insulin as a result of magnesium supplements. Insulin requirements are lower in people with Type 1 diabetes who supplement with magnesium.

The typical American diet is high in calcium and low in magnesium. Not enough magnesium results in calcium being deposited in soft tissue and arteries, which can cause strokes, circulation and heart problems. A ratio of three magnesium to one calcium is recommended. The same thing can happen with phosphate. Phosphates tend to lower magnesium levels even further. Phosphates are found in abundance in soft drinks and many processed foods. Foods rich in magnesium include whole grains, dark green vegetables, molasses, nuts, and bone meal.

For complete blood glucose regulation, you need to take all the minerals in the proper proportions and in the most absorbable form. Tablets are not the best source of supplemental minerals. Since the process of digestion is a process of liquefaction, your body has to take a hard tablet and turn it into solution. This may not be possible due to a number of factors, such as inadequate stomach acid, stress, food allergies, and intestinal problems. To get enough minerals from your supplement source, take them in solution. When they are in a liquid solution form, your body is better able to absorb and assimilate all of them.

For many years I have used Maximum Living's MineralRich, which is a delicious liquid mineral supplement that provides all the minerals the diabetic body needs, along with biotin, and is rapidly absorbed in the body.

## VITAMIN SUPPLEMENTS

New research hints that a little-known B vitamin called biotin may nip the need for the injection needle if you have diabetes. An article in the *Annals of the New York Academy of Science* reports on a study in which seven insulin-dependent diabetics were removed from insulin therapy and instead treated with 16 milligrams per day of biotin or a placebo for one week. The diabetics who received nothing saw their diabetes return, while those given the biotin saw their blood glucose level drop.

Japanese researchers found that study participants taking biotin and the glucose-lowering drug glibenclamide were able to cut their drug dosage by as much as half. The group that was taking biotin long term saw the most benefits. Within two months, glucose levels fell to nearly half their original levels.

Vitamin B6, pyridoxine, is another B vitamin found to be important to glucose metabolism. A vitamin B6 deficiency is known to reduce pancreatic and circulating insulin levels, and degenerative changes have been noted in rats fed vitamin B6-deficient diets. Gestational diabetes was eliminated in pregnant women following two weeks of treatment with 100 milligrams per day of B6 and is associated with decreased retinopathy, a common diabetes complication. Taken together, all of the evidence shows a vitamin B6 deficiency could be very important to preventing as well as reversing the diabetic condition.

For the best source of B vitamin supplements, choose Maximum Living's Vita Sprout. It contains therapeutic levels of biotin and vitamin B6, along with all the B vitamins. The B-complex vitamins provide the body with energy, metabolizing fats and protein, and are necessary for the normal functioning of the nervous system, important to prevent problems common to diabetics. Vita-Sprout is naturally sourced, using freeze-dried sprouts, vegetables, and herbs. And to make sure the entire complex of B vitamins are digested and assimilated properly, it includes friendly-body bacteria acidophilus. Nothing could be more complete for your immune system team than this power-packed, God-given formula.

People with diabetes have a higher than usual need for vitamin E, which improves insulin activity and acts as an antioxidant and a blood oxygenator. Research has shown that people with low blood levels of vitamin E are more likely to develop Type 2 diabetes. Double-blind studies show that vitamin E improves glucose tolerance in people with Type 2 diabetes and glucose tolerance in elderly non-diabetics.

The most impressive study on vitamin E and diabetes used a total of 1,350 international units of d-alpha tocopheryl daily, divided into three doses. Begin by taking 400 international units each morning. After two weeks, add another dose of 400 international units in the evening. After two more weeks, add another 400 international units in the afternoon. It may require three months or more of supplementation for benefits to become apparent. The trace mineral selenium works with vitamin E, so don't forget the MineralRich.

If you have high blood pressure, limit your intake of supplemental vitamin E to a total of 400 international units daily. If you are taking an anti-coagulant (blood thinner), consult your nutrition-minded physician before taking supplemental vitamin E.

For your supplemental vitamin E, choose Maximum Living's E-400. It uses soybean oil, a high quality natural vegetable source, for its d-alpha tocopheryl and contains no additives to diminish its potency.

Type 1 diabetics have low vitamin C levels. Vitamin C lowers sorbitol in diabetics. Sorbitol is a sugar that can accumulate and damage the eyes, nerves, and kidneys of diabetics. Vitamin C can improve glucose tolerance in Type 2 diabetes.

Insulin is one way vitamin C is transported into cells. It has been theorized that, due to impaired transport or dietary insufficiency, a relative vitamin C deficiency exists in the diabetic, and that this may be responsible for some of the circulation problems that occur in diabetics. If you are diabetic, supplement your diet with 1 to 3 grams (1,000 to 3,000 milligrams) per day of vitamin C.

Maximum Living's Solu-C (vitamin C) formulas include bioflavonoids for a one-two punch against the oxidation that leads to heart and vascular disease. Products include a tasty chewable for fast and efficient absorption and easy-to-swallow capsules that contain green tea for immune boosting and rutin, a bioflavonoid found naturally in food that is credited with strengthening the tiny capillaries of the body—important to prevent retinopathy. Rutin also helps the body assimilate vitamin C. Add the Solu-C powder to fresh fruit or juice to keep it from browning. When you pack a fresh-cut fruit salad in your lunch, mix in Solu-C powder for all day freshness and nutrition.

## BEYOND SUPPLEMENTS

Supplements are beneficial in treating the problems that occur because of diabetes: heart disease and strokes, kidney disease, retinopathy, nerve disease, arteriosclerosis, damage to the nervous system, high blood pressure, and oral infections. In the next chapters, I will isolate what diabetics can do to prevent and combat these secondary problems.

CHAPTER FIVE

# HEART HELP

*The heart of a fool is in his mouth, but the mouth of the wise man is in his heart.*

*—Benjamin Franklin*

**DIABETES AND HEART DISEASE** does not leave the well-known and well-loved free from its clutches. Recently it was reported that America's darling, Elizabeth Taylor, a diabetic, is living with congestive heart failure. I know Elizabeth personally, and I'm sorry to say she is not well.

According to an article in *The Hollywood Star,* the 73-year-old is reportedly sleeping between 12 and 14 hours a day and hasn't left her swanky Bel Air home for a month. The article quotes a friend of the actress as saying: "Elizabeth asked me what I thought heaven was going to be like. She couldn't wait to go there. With tears in her eyes she told me, 'I won't hurt anymore. I'll be with Richard (Burton).' That's all she really cares about."

Other famous females with diabetes include Halle Berry, Ella Fitzgerald, Mae West, and Winnie

Mandela. Their male counterparts include Sir Steven Redgrave, John Prescott, Chris Rea, Miles Davis, and Neil Young.

The famous writer H. G. Wells founded the British Diabetes Association in 1934, which is now Diabetes UK. Welsh singer Sir Harry Secombe has been the president for 18 years.

## HEART DISEASE—NOT A DIABETES DEATH SENTENCE

Approximately 65 percent of deaths among people with diabetes are due to heart disease and stroke—the leading cause of death among diabetics. And the risk for stroke and heart disease is two to four times higher among people with diabetes.

However, while diabetes probably does increase the odds of having and dying from heart disease, the people who represent these numbers were probably depending wholly on medications to control their condition. I'd like to see statistics on people who use diet, exercise, and nutritional supplementation. The numbers would be drastically lower.

There is much you can do to minimize, and even reverse, the damage to the cardiovascular system caused by excessive and fluctuating blood glucose.

Here's a review of what we've already covered:

- Eat foods with a low Glycemic Index.
- Eat foods high in fiber.
- Eat whole grains and fresh raw vegetables and fruit.
- Avoid processed, fatty, and preserved foods.

- Get moderate regular exercise (you will lose weight over time so hang in there).

One newly discovered factor causing heart problems isn't a surprise for those of us who have seen what works and what doesn't. The nutrients that do the most good in the fight against heart disease also happen to fight inflammation. Studies in the past few years have shown that inflammation plays a vital role in arteriosclerosis, the buildup of fatty deposits in blood vessels that can lead to heart attacks, strokes, and other cardiovascular problems.

It's not surprising that foods that contain anti-inflammatory nutrients are eaten among cultures and countries that have the lowest rates of heart disease. Interesting to note is that the healthiest populations are those who maintain the diet of their ancestors—indigenous food—and that in order to recover health, cultures are moving back to the old ways of eating.

Many of the spices and flavorings traditionally used in the zesty cuisine of East India and Thailand are heart healthy. They include tamarind, tumeric, garlic, cinnamon, clove, cardamom, lemon grass, chili peppers, and ginger.

## EAT MEDITERRANEAN

Mediterranean cuisine is also renowned. Many think it is the best in the world. People in the countries around the Mediterranean Sea revel in their food and wine and spend long hours preparing and eating a variety of delicious dishes. Food is an integral part of their culture, yet they have one of the lowest rates of heart disease for any population in the world.

A recent study found that men with slightly higher than normal blood pressure were much more likely to die of coronary heart disease if they lived in the United States and northern Europe rather than Mediterranean southern Europe.

The Mediterranean diet is mainly vegetarian—rich in olive oil, fruits, garlic, vegetables, and whole grains, and low in meat, dairy products, and sweet desserts. The foods typically eaten are low in cholesterol and high in vitamins, anti-inflammatory flavonoids, minerals, and polyunsaturated fats.

Onions, garlic, and tomatoes, surrounded by olive oil, begin many dishes. Eggplants abound, as do squashes, peppers, mushrooms, cucumbers, artichokes, okra, and various greens and lettuces. Legumes too are plentiful: lentils, chick peas, fava beans, green beans, and white kidney beans. Fresh herbs include rosemary, basil, cilantro, parsley, mint, dill, fennel, and oregano.

Seafood remains at the core of the Mediterranean cooking heritage. All manner of shellfish is eaten in soups, stews, and pastas. Anchovies, fresh and cured, are widely eaten, as are various white-fleshed fish, such as sole, flounder, and grouper. Other seafood served in the region include swordfish, monkfish, eel, cuttlefish, squid, and octopus.

Beef is rare in Mediterranean cuisine, for the land cannot support large herds. Smaller animals, such as lamb, goats, sheep, pork, rabbit, and fowl, provide most of the meat. Sheep and goats provide dairy for enzyme-rich yogurts and cheeses.

Olive oil, rich in cholesterol-lowering fatty acids, is essential for any heart-smart diet. But not all olive oils are the same. The longer an oil is on the shelf, the less nutrients it contains. The freshest olive oils contain the most vitamins and the most concentration of essential fatty acids. My olive oil comes straight from the orchard. I use Villa Mille Rose Extra Virgin Olive Oil from Napa Valley, California. I love its taste, and even more, I love what it does for my cardiovascular system. To order this wonderful oil, write to: 1090 Chestnut Street #10, San Francisco, CA 94109; phone: 415-673-6800; oliveoil@villamillerose.com.

## MORE HEART-SMART FOODS

*Eat fish.* It's the oil in fish that makes it so heart healthy. Fish oil is an omega-3 fatty acid. In areas where fish consumption is high, such as Japan, Greenland, and the Mediterranean, people eat considerably more fish than in the U.S. They also have a much lower risk for cardiovascular disease. Fish with the highest amounts of omega-3 are: Atlantic mackerel, albacore tuna, Atlantic herring, Chinook salmon, lake trout, Atlantic salmon, and bluefin tuna. I recommend you eat fish two to three times a week.

*Eat berries.* Colorful foods, such as berries, have the highest amounts of flavonoids, substances proven to reduce the inflammation that can turn cholesterol into a stroke. Berries contain the most, but flavonoids are also present in colorful fruits and vegetables. Do you have allergies? One study found that flavonoids effectively reduce the histamine reaction common in allergy reactions.

*Appreciate garlic.* Garlic acts as a natural chelator, thinning the blood and pushing fats and toxins out of the bloodstream. The ancient Greeks used garlic to keep the arteries open. Garlic eaten with a fatty meal will dramatically reduce cholesterol and fat levels in the blood. When taken for a couple of months, garlic can drop the level of cholesterol in the blood by 15 percent. Just half a clove of garlic a day thins the blood and reduces the stickiness that can contribute to plaque buildup. Garlic only works when raw (or supplemented). Try chopped raw garlic in Chinese ginger salad or try pickled garlic.

*Eat onions and apples.* A Dutch study found that men who ate the most food containing flavonoids, such as apples and onions, suffered half as many fatal heart attacks as men who consumed the lowest amounts. Men who had a higher intake of flavonoids had a lower risk of death from coronary heart disease and of having a first heart attack. Onions and apple peel contain quercetin, a flavonoid credited with reducing inflammation.

*Eat grapes.* Grapes contain potent flavonoids. The people of the Mediterranean drink a lot of red wine. I don't advocate alcohol, but in one study non-wine drinkers had one-third more heart problems than low to moderate drinkers. Get the flavonoids without the alcohol by eating red or black grapes or drinking grape juice.

*Appreciate spicy food.* Cayenne pepper, tumeric, and ginger are all noted for their health-giving properties. Turmeric has been used in both the Indian and Chinese systems of medicine (and their food) for the treatment of many forms of inflammation.

*Become a vegetarian.* Not only are fruits, grains, and vegetables better for you, too much high protein meat increases cholesterol. Researchers found that when people ate a high protein diet for a year, blood vessel inflammation jumped 62 percent and coronary artery disease worsened. If you can't do without meat, choose animals that have been range fed. Grass contains omega-3 fatty acids while corn does not.

While I'm at it, *don't cook meat on high heat.* If you broil, make it fish. Grilling, broiling, and frying meat and poultry create damaged proteins called AGEs (advanced glycosylation end products) that trigger inflammation. In diabetics who ate a high AGE-inducing diet, inflammation jumped 35 percent. Mount Sinai School of Medicine researchers discovered it dropped 20 percent in those on low AGE-inducing diets. To reduce AGEs, poach or boil chicken, and eat more fish. Broiled fish has about one-fourth the AGEs of broiled steak or chicken. Fruits and vegetables are low in AGEs; cheeses are high in them.

## HEART-SMART SUPPLEMENTS

There are certain nutritional supplements that benefit the heart and blood vessels. These include nutrients that thin the blood so it flows smoothly, nutrients that strengthen the blood vessels so they withstand blood pressure fluctuations, and nutrients that strengthen heart muscles so blood pumps efficiently and consistently. Thankfully all are available to consumers in this country.

"There is growing recognition that the relationship between diet and heart disease needs to be broadened to include not only dietary fat and cholesterol, but also dietary sources of vitamins, which may protect against heart disease and stroke," said Dr. Irwin H. Rosenberg, professor of physiology, medicine, and nutrition at Tufts University.

A Canadian survey of over 2,200 men found that those who had been taking vitamins of any kind reduced the risk of death from heart disease by 78 percent, cut their risk of a heart attack by 58 percent, and reduced their risk of angina (spasm of the coronary artery) by 15 percent.

### *B Vitamins*

Probably the most recent nutritional find is the connection between the B vitamins and the risk of heart problems. The connection began as researchers discovered that high levels of homocysteine—a naturally occurring amino acid in the blood—increases the risk of heart disease, and vitamins B12, B6, and folic acid help regulate levels of homocysteine.

### *Magnesium*

For the past 50 years, doctors have successfully used magnesium in the treatment of cardiac arrhythmia. This was in response to numerous uncontrolled studies and to the knowledge that it doesn't cause side effects.

A deficiency of magnesium can cause heart problems. When people with cardiovascular problems and low magnesium intake try to improve their health with strenuous exercise, such as jogging, they could be endangering their health. Magnesium requirements are markedly increased during physical stress, and the heart is much more susceptible to arrhythmia during physical exertion if the body's magnesium level is low.

During my television show, *Making Healthy Choices*, Michael Schachter, M.D., agreed, stating that many cases of sudden heart attacks during stressful exercise can be directly attributed to a magnesium deficiency.

Important to remember is that magnesium must be balanced with calcium and potassium for the proper regulation of heart muscle contraction. Take all the minerals together, in solution, for the most efficient use by the body of all of them.

### *Antioxidants*

Antioxidants work in virtually all aspects of heart disease. They help blood circulation, inhibit blood platelets from sticking together, and reduce plaque in the arteries. Many studies show that antioxidant vitamins may reduce the risk of coronary artery disease.

A study at the University of Southern California School of Medicine found that heart patients who took 100 IU of vitamin E plus niacin had fewer heart problems over two years than those who did not take the vitamins. The Physicians Health Study showed vitamin E protected patients against heart disease.

In the Scottish Heart Health Study, over 10,000 middle-aged men were evaluated for their intakes of vitamins C, E, and beta carotene. It was found that these antioxidants had a highly protective effect on their hearts.

One kind of heart problem has been directly linked to a deficiency of the mineral selenium, a particularly potent antioxidant. Keshan's disease was first discovered in Keshan County in the Heilongjiang Province of China, where it was rampant in 1935. Once it was discovered that selenium deficiency was the underlying cause of the disease and selenium supplementation could prevent it, it stopped being a major public health problem.

Copper and zinc are two minerals noted for their antioxidant and healing properties. They work together, and a deficiency of one will create a deficiency in the other.

Another antioxidant proven to help the heart is coenzyme Q10, a nutrient found in studies to help fight congestive heart failure (CHF), a common condition where the heart becomes too weak to pump enough blood to the tissues of the body.

Flavonoids, found in many vegetables, fruits, and berries, are active in the fight against arterial insufficiency. As antioxidants, they prevent the deterioration of blood vessels by free radicals, retard inflammation resulting from cellular damage that can contribute to narrowing, and smooth artery walls.

Probably the most potent flavonoid discovered by researchers is ginkgo biloba. When extracted from the plant and concentrated, it has been shown in studies to be far superior to pentoxifylline, the pharmaceutical treatment of choice for people suffering from intermittent claudication (a cramping pain, induced by exercise, that is caused by inadequate blood supply in the affected muscles).

Out of nine double-blind randomized clinical trials of ginkgo biloba versus a placebo in patients with diminished leg circulation, all found it to be of significant benefit. Ginkgo biloba, while being poo-pooed by the FDA in the United States, is now among the leading prescription medicines in Germany and France. The extracts account for 1 percent and 1.5 percent of total prescription sales in Germany and France, respectively. Fortunately, those in need in the U.S. can get it wherever health food items are sold.

## MAXIMIZE YOUR HEALTH WITH MAXIMUM LIVING

Maximum Living has several products rich in flavonoids and antioxidants.

Solu-C mimics the healthiest natural food by matching citrus flavonoids with natural vitamin C.

Ginkgo biloba with DHA includes the flavonoid terpene derived from the leaves of the ginkgo biloba tree. DHA is an omega-3 fatty acid essential to the nervous system, important to the health of anyone with diabetes.

Of course, there's Maximum Living's E-400, the best source of natural antioxidant vitamin E on the market.

Maximum Living also makes a power-packed antioxidant formula, containing the best antioxidants from a variety of sources: mineral, vitamin, amino acid, and herbal. It includes the aforementioned diabetic-healthy antioxidants: ginkgo biloba, chromium, selenium, zinc, copper, vitamin C, vitamin E, and others. It is your first source for a comprehensive antioxidant formula.

For an excellent natural source of coenzyme Q10, choose the Maximum Living formula. It includes vitamin E, selenium, and phospholipids from lecithin, which help assimilate cholesterol so it doesn't accumulate in arteries and dissolve scar tissue so it doesn't cause blockages.

While you're eating fish, supplement with the essential fatty acid contained in it. Maximum Living's flaxseed oil contains the vegetable version of fish oil and a better source of omega-3 fatty acids. And, unlike fish, it has a better shelf life, doesn't need to be refrigerated, and isn't risked by chemical pollutants.

Maximum Living also offers an excellent aged garlic extract formula that concentrates all the heart-beneficial agents of garlic into a form easy to take and even better for health. It is odorless too, so you don't have to worry that you'll lose your friends and acquaintances.

For your best source of B vitamins, don't forget Maximum Living's Vita Sprout. Derived from 1/4" alfalfa seed sprouts, the natural basis of this formula ensures optimal assimilation and potency.

For more on maintaining heart health and overcoming problems, read my booklet, *Super Heart Health*.

## CONTROL YOUR BLOOD PRESSURE

Another complication common to people with diabetes is high blood pressure, so in the next chapter I will show you how you can monitor and control your blood pressure without dangerous pharmaceutical drugs.

CHAPTER SIX

# HYPERTENSION AND KIDNEY DISEASE

*Old age is when you resent the swimsuit issue of Sports Illustrated because there are fewer articles to read.*

*—George Burns*

**IN HIS LAST YEARS GEORGE BURNS** was known for being old, yet alert and active, and was often seen on the arm of a buxom Hollywood starlet. His jokes were corny and self-effacing. When asked why he didn't date women his age, he said there weren't any. The fact that he retained his wit and energy and still lived to be 100 can likely be attributed to his sense of humor.

If anyone can be called a healer, it is the comedian. This is because laughter truly is medicinal. Laughter produces endorphins, the body's natural painkillers. Hearty laughter is literally good for the heart, because when we laugh it causes our blood vessels to dilate.

An important part of taking care of yourself is keeping your blood pressure under control. High blood pressure—also called hypertension—raises your risk for heart attack, stroke, eye problems, and kidney disease. High blood pressure is estimated to affect 20 to 60 percent of diabetics, depending on obesity, ethnicity, and age. In Type 2 diabetes, hypertension can mean the breakdown of the kidneys. In Type 1 diabetes, hypertension may mean the beginning of nervous system damage.

My first recommendation for blood pressure control is laughter. Whatever you enjoy, bring it on. Experiments have proved that there is a drop of 10 to 20 mm. in blood pressure after participating in a 10-minute laughter session. Laughter also helps in stopping the further progress of heart disease as it improves blood circulation and oxygen supply to the heart muscles. Due to improvement of blood circulation, there are less chances of forming a clot.

## HIGH BLOOD PRESSURE

Blood pressure is the force of blood flow inside your blood vessels. When your blood moves through your vessels with too much force, you have high blood pressure. Your heart has to work harder when blood pressure is high, and your risk for diabetes problems increases.

Both diabetes and high blood pressure increase your risk of heart attack, stroke, and eye and kidney disease. Because of this, people with diabetes have a lower blood pressure target than the general public (less than 130/80).

Hypertension is often called the "quiet killer" for the reason that it doesn't always show signs of the damage it may be doing: 1) weakening blood vessel walls; 2) aneurysms—abnormal expanding or hazardous ballooning of the artery wall, which, when ruptured, can cause strokes, heart attacks, or instant death; and 3) congestive heart failure and kidney damage.

## THE MINERAL ALLIANCE

One of the most common conventional treatments for hypertension is calcium-channel blockers. These drugs are supposed to attach to the surface membrane of the muscles in the artery walls and prevent calcium from entering. The drugs are also prescribed for the treatment of coronary artery disease or heart-rhythm abnormalities.

What doctors don't tell you is that magnesium does what these drugs do, but better.

Probably the most beneficial nutritional discovery of our time is the finding that magnesium is a calcium-channel blocker, and it strengthens veins and arteries. Researchers found that in the blood cells of laboratory rats, a lack of magnesium resulted in higher amounts of calcium, and that when there were high amounts of calcium in the cells, they became inactive and ineffective.

## WATCH THE SALT

Sodium is a mineral, which the average American eats too much of, thanks to its prolific use in food processing and preservation. While it is obvious at this point we're better off without so much preserved and salted food, it is a lack of the other minerals that causes the damage. When it comes to sodium and hypertension, potassium and magnesium are the missing factors.

Eating too much salt will not cause high blood pressure. But if you don't get enough potassium in your diet and eat too much salt, you'll be risking it. It is no longer acceptable to recommend lowering salt (sodium chloride) intake alone. First calcium, potassium, and magnesium deficits should be corrected. The evidence suggests salt would not be a factor if these minerals were present in sufficient quantities. Also, low magnesium appears to cause or have a connection with low potassium.

If you are hypertensive, cut down on salt and eat foods high in potassium. Eliminate soft drinks. They rob your body of potassium.

## SUGAR AND HYPERTENSION

There is no doubt in my mind that today's typical American eating habits are killing us. Consider these statistics: 46 percent of every food dollar is spent on meals and snacks away from home. Convenience stores have increased by 50 percent over the last decade. The typical American consumes 48 pounds of high fructose corn syrup annually—mostly in soft drinks. No wonder America is experiencing an epidemic of degenerative diseases! With these habits, who needs auto accidents?

In a study of hypertensive rats, it took only two weeks on a high sugar diet for the rats to see a marked increase in their blood pressure, and this effect could be turned off and on just with the addition of sugar in their diets. Richard A. Ahrens, Ph.D., of the University of Maryland's College of Human Ecology, found the same results in humans, concluding that sugar contributes to sodium retention.

If you are diabetic and have high blood pressure, supplement with MineralRich, avoid processed and salty foods and sugary snacks, and maybe you won't have problems with your kidneys. But just in case…

## KIDNEY DISEASE

Diabetes is the most common cause of kidney failure, accounting for more than 40 percent of new cases. However, that still leaves 60 percent of people with diabetes who do not develop kidney disease (diabetic nephropathy) severe enough to cause kidney failure. Of the approximate 18 million diabetics in the United States, over 100,000 people are living with kidney failure as a result of it.

Hope for the best but prepare for the worst. Since an early diagnosis of kidney disease is important, know the signs:

- Increased or decreased urination
- Blood in urine
- Flank pain (i.e., pain that radiates from the side to the lower back)

- Puffiness or swelling of the extremities (legs, feet, arms, hands) or face
- Excessively itchy skin
- Unexplained fatigue
- Shortness of breath
- Unexplained feelings of being cold
- Nausea and vomiting
- Difficulty concentrating
- Unexplained weight loss
- Decreased appetite

**INDIGENOUS FOODS**

African Americans, American Indians, and Hispanic Americans develop diabetes, nephropathy, and kidney failure at rates higher than average. Scientists have not been able to explain these higher rates, but I suspect it is because these cultures are adopting diets alien to the foods of their ancestors.

In the American Southwest, the Pima and the Tohono O'odham Native American tribes are throwing off the diabetes sickness by discarding fast foods and the convenient, more sedentary ways of the modern world and returning to the seeds, nuts, berries, beans, and corns of their ancestral diet.

If you look at the typical American diet, you can identify the poisons that infect the blood, heart, kidneys, and eyes of the diabetic. The main poison is fatty meat. Beef, as we know it today, was not eaten by anyone's ancestors. Early cattle were used for milk and labor and weren't eaten until they became too old to work. In the most ancient of civilizations, cattle were not eaten at all.

**EAT LESS MEAT**

We've been trained to believe that a meal is not a meal without meat. In restaurants even the salads have meat. So it isn't surprising that the first course of action when a kidney is in jeopardy is to cut down on meat protein.

Research shows that by lowering the amount of protein intake the risk of end stage renal disease, i.e. reaching the need for dialysis, can be reduced by 30 percent in diabetic patients.

Amino acid supplements have shown promise in treating chronic renal failure, when coupled with a greatly restricted amount of meat protein of only 20 to 25 grams a day (one ounce). As an advocate of vegetable juice fasting, I personally think the protein restriction may have accomplished as much as the amino acid supplementation. Why? Because a typical hospital "protein restricted diet" provides 40 grams per day of protein!

Consider this: the typical American eats over 100 grams and frequently exceeds 120 grams of meat protein daily, which is WAY too much. So a so-called "restriction" to 40 grams per day is simply a correction. Most of the world's people would be pleased as punch to be able to eat 40 grams of meat a day. But we happily chow down three times that, call it "normal," and then line up for dialysis.

A low protein diet for people who have kidney disease, but not failure, should consist of 0.6 grams of protein per day per kilogram of body weight. This translates roughly into 2 ounces of meat per day for a 200-pound man or 1-1/2 ounces of meat for a 150-pound woman.

Remember, I'm talking about meat here. Doctors caution against protein restriction because we need protein to thrive. But complex carbohydrates can be eaten for protein—the kind of protein that doesn't acidify the blood and create excess phosphorus, jeopardizing the kidneys. In order to get complete protein in one meal, you simply have to combine them properly.

To reach your daily allowance of complete protein combine whole grains with legumes. The Greek dish felafel combines whole wheat pita bread with garbanzo beans. Latin Americans get their protein by combining corn tortillas with beans. In India, it's rice or wheat chapatis with lentils. Other protein plant food combinations are nuts and seeds with legumes, and nuts and seeds with dark green leafy vegetables. Eat a green salad with kidney beans and sunflower seeds. There you have it: a good source of protein and lots of other essential nutrients! Beats a steak any day.

Maximum Living makes an amino acid formula that is more therapeutic than the average. It contains free form amino acids, as well as those typically left out of health maintenance formulas. Just because most people don't always need certain nutrients doesn't mean they shouldn't be included. Maximum Living formulas are not based on Recommended Daily Allowances for healthy people; they are designed for those who need more to overcome illness.

## ANTIOXIDANT VITAMINS C AND E

Untreated, diabetes raises blood pressure and increases the production of damaging oxidizing agents called free radicals. Free radicals convert sugar and protein into chemicals that damage body tissues and organs.

Researchers found that when they added vitamins C and E to insulin, this damaging conversion was prevented, thus protecting the kidneys, eyes, and nervous system.

There is a nasty rumor that vitamin C causes kidney stones, which is not true. Rather, vitamin C increases urine flow and favorably lowers the pH to help keep stones from forming. In fact, the vitamin has been used since the late 1940s to prevent and treat kidney stones.

Vitamin C is a potent antioxidant, and this is why it prevents not only kidney stones, but kidney damage related to diabetes. It can mean the difference between a weak kidney and one damaged beyond repair.

Vitamin C is a water-soluble vitamin, which means the body excretes what it doesn't use. In order to achieve the most optimal benefit, it has to be in the system at all times. This is accomplished most readily by establishing a bowel tolerance dosage. Begin by taking 1,000 milligrams every hour until you notice a little diarrhea. Cut the dosage to just below that and take a third that amount three times a day, so the bowel tolerance amount is taken three times a day.

Remember that the best form of vitamin C contains food-derived flavonoids, such as Maximum Living's Solu-C.

Vitamin E is not water soluble, so I recommend 400 milligrams a day of Maximum Living's vitamin E formula. You can trust it for your antioxidant needs.

## PROTECTING THE EYES

In the next chapter, I'll talk more about antioxidants in relation to another diabetic challenge: retinopathy, a general term for all disorders of the eye's retina caused by the diabetic condition.

CHAPTER SEVEN

# RETINOPATHY AND CHOLESTEROL

*He that is strucken blind cannot forget the precious treasure of his eyesight lost.*

*—William Shakespeare*

**"I'M HAVING TROUBLE SEEING,"** Bob said to his friend, blinking his eyes intentionally, as though that might help. "My vision is cloudy, and I've given up driving for fear I won't see oncoming cars." His friend drew a deep breath, knowing that Bob's diabetes could be affecting his eyesight.

Consider what it would be like to not be able to look into your loved one's eyes…or to behold crimson and gold canopies on an autumn day…or to gaze up into the universe on a clear night and behold the heavens. Our eyesight is a precious gift from God that enables us to experience the wonder of the world in which we live. Clear eyesight gives us the ability to walk confidently, to drive, to read, and to continue doing the things that we love.

All is not lost. Help is at hand. But to uncover the solutions you must first understand how and why the problems occur.

According to the American Diabetes Association, diabetic retinopathy is a general term for all disorders of the retina caused by diabetes. What it means to the diabetic is that he or she has been unsuccessful in controlling blood sugar levels, and the disease has started to break down the body.

In the early stages of retinopathy, the tiny capillaries in the eyes balloon to form pouches. Although vision loss does not occur at this stage, the capillary walls may lose their ability to control the passage of substances between the blood and the retina. As a result, the retina becomes swollen and fatty deposits form within it. If this swelling affects the center of the retina, the problem is called macular edema. This can cause some vision loss.

In later stages, the blood vessels are so damaged that they close off. In response, new blood vessels start growing in the retina. These new vessels are weak and can leak blood, blocking vision, a condition called vitreous hemorrhage. The damage can also cause scar tissue to grow. When the scar tissue shrinks, it can distort the retina or pull it out of place (retinal detachment). The worst part is, the retina can be damaged before a person notices any symptoms or changes in vision.

According to conventional medicine, the longer a person has diabetes, the more likely they are to have retinopathy. It is estimated that after 60 years, 98 percent of diabetics will have some form of retinopathy, 42 percent will have macular edema, and 28 percent will experience severe vision loss. This is not your prediction. These figures are based on subjects who probably do not have the information contained in this booklet.

The good news is that even severe cases of retinopathy can regress and vision can improve through diet and supplements.

## ANTIOXIDANTS FOR DIABETIC EYES

You should be familiar with the term *free radical* by now. All you need to know is that it occurs over time, is worsened by oxygen and chemicals, and effectively destroys your body tissues, including the delicate eye tissues. Cholesterol, or fat, can increase free radical damage.

Fat, whether clogging your drain pipes, your heart arteries, or your eye capillaries, not only obstructs circulation but invites bacteria, which feed on it and produce vile acids. These acids encourage free radical damage.

High cholesterol can contribute to diabetic retinopathy. Japanese researchers conducted a study of 104 non-insulin dependent diabetic patients. They found that those with high cholesterol levels were more at risk for retinopathy.

Dietary fat is such an important factor in

retinopathy that patients have reversed the disorder just by eating less of it. In one study, 64 percent of 44 retinopathy patients showed improvement after going on a low fat diet. Impressive alone, but eight of the patients eventually saw their retinopathy completely disappear.

This would explain the studies that show antioxidants—nutrients that reverse the oxidative, free radical damage of fat and cholesterol—help reverse diabetic retinopathy.

A preliminary trial conducted by researchers at Hoffman-La Roche & Co. found the antioxidants beta carotene, vitamins C and E, and selenium not only helped stop the retinal degeneration of diabetic patients, but in some cases reversed the damage.

In a Japanese study, researchers gave 90 to 180 milligrams of vitamin E daily to 38 patients with diabetic retinopathy. After 19 to 24 months on this therapy, 67 percent of all patients reported significant improvement in their condition.

Some eye doctors believe vitamin E helps treat a detached retina. For retinal nerve hemorrhages, Gershon M. Lesser, M.D., has found vitamins A, C, and E, along with zinc and omega-3, useful.

## SEE BETTER WITH VITAMIN C AND FLAVONOIDS

Anthocyanosides are a class of flavonoids found in fruits and vegetables, most notably blueberries, grapes, and bilberries. They are known for their anti-inflammatory, oxygen-quenching, antioxidant, and tissue-enhancement properties.

Aldose reductase is an enzyme believed to be the culprit in the damaging effect of diabetes. Aldose reductase transforms excess blood sugar into an alcohol sugar the body can't burn, and this accumulates in nerve cells and damages them. Researchers have found one flavonoid that not only reverses free radical damage, reduces inflammation, and boosts tissue health, but inhibits the accumulation of aldose reductase. Call it the diabetic friend. Call it quercetin. It is available in health food stores, vitamin formulas, and in apples, citrus fruit, and yellow and red onions.

In some cases, retinopathy occurs when the delicate capillaries of the eyes aren't strong enough to avoid hemorrhaging and leaking, leading some researchers to contend it is not high blood pressure as much as poor capillary strength that causes retinopathy and loss of the retina. Studying what could reverse this, researchers hit on vitamin C and flavonoids—rutin from buckwheat, most specifically—as compounds that strengthen capillaries and prevent leaking.

In a case history, a 72-year-old woman with sudden loss of vision in her left eye experienced dramatic restoration of vision with rutin. Doctors noted in the *American Journal of Ophthalmology* that 75 percent of cases of capillary leakage can be restored to normal by using 500 milligrams a day of rutin, and that rutin universally improves capillary strength, stops the progression of retinopathy, and benefits diabetics in general.

Another flavonoid found effective in preventing or reversing retinopathy is catechin, found in green tea leaves. Quercetin and catechin are both free radical fighters and, when combined with vitamin C, create the best offense and defense teams. In one study, researchers noted that guinea pigs given low levels of vitamin C showed the same blood levels as those not given vitamin C—until they were also given catechin—then the levels shot up.

Researchers have been studying ginkgo's flavonoid power to increase blood flow through aging capillaries, especially in the eyes. Its ability to increase circulation and reduce inflammation gives it high marks for resolving eye problems. The flavonoids in gingko biloba leaves help keep the heart, veins, and arteries healthy, strengthening and enlarging the vein to allow a freer flow of blood. Ginkgo was given to diabetic rats for two months, and there was a noticeable protective effect against deterioration of the retina. Ginkgo has been used by the Chinese medicinally for centuries to treat their aged.

Because of their ability to fight free radicals, reduce inflammation, and strengthen capillaries, flavonoids are literally the "finger in the dike" of diabetic retinopathy. They are the blue and red pigments found in plums, berries, apples, grapes, red onions, and pomegranates. They are the citrus rind of oranges, grapefruits, and lemons. And they are the chlorophyll in dark green vegetables and leaves.

## THE GOOD FATS

In recent years, researchers have learned that an omega-3 fatty acid, docosahexaenoic acid (DHA), is the most prominent polyunsaturated fat in the retina, and that a lack of it in the diabetic diet may contribute to retinopathy. Ironically, chronically high blood sugar in diabetics blocks an enzyme that processes omega-3 from food sources into DHA, so supplemental forms are necessary.

Omega-3 and omega-6 fatty acids also help assimilate cholesterol in the body, so it doesn't accumulate in tissues, veins, and arteries. You can find omega-3 in flaxseed oil, cod liver oil, and in cold water fish, such as trout, mackerel, sardines, tuna, and eel. Omega-3 fatty acids are also found in fresh dark green vegetables, such as broccoli, kale, collards, and Swiss chard.

Also found to benefit is omega-6 fatty acids, most especially borage oil, which contains the highest amount of gamma linolenic acid (GLA). Very large doses of GLA have been shown to reduce by two-thirds the risk of eye disease over a period of about six years.

## MAGNANIMOUS MINERALS

Low blood levels of the mineral magnesium is also associated with diabetic retinopathy. A medical journal reported that diabetic retinopathy patients have the lowest magnesium levels, and that supplementing with magnesium can help diabetic patients reduce the damaging effect of their condition.

Once again, we have a connection to cholesterol and heart disease. Doctors use magnesium injections to counter high blood pressure, strokes, and heart disease. It works by dilating the capillaries so blood runs faster and smoother and can pull out cholesterol deposits. It's also important for circulation and blockages, *and* sufficient amounts are needed to convert blood sugar into energy.

A mineral secret is copper for high cholesterol. Supplementing with copper can lower cholesterol 800 times more than saturated fat has been shown to raise it. Symptoms of a copper deficiency include heart palpitations, fatigue, depression, *and* high cholesterol.

Magnesium is nature's calcium traffic cop, directing calcium to the parts of the body where it is needed and making sure it doesn't go where it doesn't belong. Since every tissue in the diabetic's body is shown to have increased levels of calcium, magnesium is essential so that calcium doesn't contribute to blockages.

## CHOLESTEROL LOWERERS

While it is true that otherwise healthy individuals can live with high cholesterol, because of the delicate nature of the diabetic system, maintaining lower levels of cholesterol is important. Fortunately, medications aren't necessary because there are many foods and nutrients capable of doing just that. It's easier to depend on nutrition and much less risky.

Fiber can reduce cholesterol levels. Certain kinds of fiber, particularly, have been shown to help. Australian researchers found that adult rats fed oat bran lowered cholesterol levels better than wheat bran. Psyllium is another source of fiber that has been found in many studies to lower LDL cholesterol by as much as 39 percent.

Beans, peas, and lentils contain fiber that helps the colon and lowers blood cholesterol. A cup of pinto or navy beans eaten every day was found to lower cholesterol by 19 percent.

Yams or sweet potatoes contain much water-soluble fiber, as well as beta carotene, a potent antioxidant that prevents the fats in your body from eating away your insides. Consumed four or five times weekly, yams will contribute to a program of cholesterol control. Japanese researchers rated the fiber in sweet potatoes as best of 28 fruit and vegetable fibers for binding with cholesterol and removing it.

It isn't coincidence that vegetarians typically have lower blood cholesterol than their meat-eating counterparts. If you don't depend on meat for your entrees, you'll be amazed at the variety of health-giving food from which you can choose. From A to Z, cholesterol-lowering foods are: apples, almonds, avocados, bananas, barley, beans, chili peppers, eggplant, garlic, fruit pectin, oat bran, olive oil, onions, kelp, lentils, peas, green plantains, soybeans, spinach, sweet potatoes, walnuts, yams, and yogurt with active cultures.

Soybeans and the products derived from them, such as soy milk, lecithin, and tofu, help break down fatty deposits so they can be flushed from the body more readily. This process also lowers cholesterol. Soybean products seem to work best on people with extra-high cholesterol—300 or more.

Slightly more than an ounce daily of lecithin—a food substance derived from soybeans—has been shown to reduce blood levels of cholesterol by 18 percent. Researchers at the University of Milan, Italy saw cholesterol levels in their subjects plummet by 15 to 20 percent, simply by having them eat soybeans used in various recipes in place of meat and milk products.

Yogurt is a real winner in lowering cholesterol. Three cups a day have caused cholesterol levels to decline by as much as 5 to 10 percent a week, with the proportion of good guy HDL rising in proportion to LDL. Beware of yogurt substitutes, however. Read the label. Many so-called yogurts are simply milk, corn sweeteners, food starch, and gelatin, among other unnatural or unhealthy ingredients. Look for yogurt with active cultures. Plain yogurt is your best bet. Use your blender to make a smoothie with it using fresh fruit.

In one study, three medium-sized raw carrots eaten daily was shown to reduce cholesterol by almost 11 percent. That must be how Bugs Bunny does it. He never ages!

Chili peppers reduce blood serum cholesterol by suppressing the liver's ability to produce cholesterol. When researchers in Bangkok, Thailand, added freshly ground jalapeno pepper to rice flour noodles, subjects who ate the noodles daily experienced lowered cholesterol and an increased ability to dissolve blood clots.

Garlic doesn't work hanging on the wall or around your neck—you have to eat it. A ration of five fresh raw cloves minced into other foods daily for 25 days has been shown to lower blood serum cholesterol by nearly 10 percent.

## RETINAL PROTECTORS AND CHOLESTEROL LOWERERS

To strengthen retinal capillaries and prevent cardiovascular complications, Maximum Living offers Ginkgo Biloba with DHA. For optimal eyesight and circulation, the ginkgo is extracted from leaves, and for additional benefit, DHA is included.

A special Maximum Living antioxidant formula was designed specifically to benefit eyesight. OptiMax contains a multitude of powerful antioxidants as well as ingredients known to boost eye health, such as bilberry and quercetin.

Solu-C includes vitamin C with the supportive flavonoids rutin and quercetin, and for omega-3 and omega-6 fatty acids and DHA, take Maximum Living's borage oil and flaxseed oil supplements.

Supplemental garlic works better than raw garlic as a cholesterol-lowering agent. Maximum Living's garlic extract also includes antioxidants.

Maximum Living's Hyssop Cleanse includes hyssop and psyllium, as well as other food-derived sources of fiber for cholesterol-lowering.

## ONE LAST SERIOUS MATTER

In the last chapter, I will discuss the reason diabetics get limbs amputated. It's called neuropathy (nervous system disease), and it can be helped.

CHAPTER EIGHT

# NEUROPATHY (NERVE DISEASE)

> ***We are the carriers of health and disease—either the divine health of courage and nobility or the demonic diseases of hate and anxiety.***
>
> —*Joshua Loth Liebman*

**YOUR NERVOUS SYSTEM IS SIMILAR** to insulated wire. As long as the insulation is intact and strong, the wires stay clean and effective. But if something eats through the insulation, the wires can corrode and touch one another, causing short circuits (pain and muscle weakness) and loss of energy (numbness).

Chronic high blood sugar, over time, corrodes the protective coating of nerves (technically called the myelin sheath), eventually causing damage to the nerves themselves. This process, which occurs over many years, is called neuropathy. The highest rates of neuropathy are among diabetics who have had the disease for at least 25 years.

## SYMPTOMS OF NEUROPATHY

Symptoms of neuropathy depend on which nerves are affected. Some people have no symptoms at all. For others, numbness, tingling, or pain in the feet is often the first sign. A person can experience both pain and numbness. Symptoms are minor at first, and since most nerve damage occurs over several years, mild cases may go unnoticed or ignored for a long time.

The most common type is peripheral neuropathy, which causes either pain or loss of feeling in the toes, feet, legs, hands, and arms.

Symptoms of any type of neuropathy can include:

- numbness or insensitivity to pain or temperature
- a tingling, burning, or prickling sensation
- sharp pains or cramps
- extreme sensitivity to touch, even a light touch
- profuse sweating at night or while eating
- loss of balance and coordination

Blisters and sores may appear on numb areas of the feet, because pressure or injury goes unnoticed. If foot injuries are not treated promptly, the infection may spread to the bone, and the foot may then have to be amputated.

## NOURISHING YOUR NERVOUS SYSTEM

Just as there is food and nutrients for the heart and vascular system, and for the kidneys and eyes, there is food and nutrients that nourish the nervous system and have been shown in studies to help reverse and diminish diabetic neuropathies.

The B-complex vitamins provide the body with energy, metabolizing fats and protein, and are necessary for the normal functioning of the nervous system. They are the single most important factor for the health of the nerves.

A deficiency of certain B vitamins is known to cause peripheral neuropathy. Symptoms of this type of neuropathy when associated with pernicious anemia (vitamin B12 deficiency) include leg and foot pain and numbness. A B6 deficiency can cause carpal tunnel syndrome (with symptoms of numbness, tingling, and pain in the hands and wrists) and degeneration of peripheral nerves.

Another reason the B vitamins are important to the nervous system is that they help break down fats/cholesterol in the body. One of the ways in which a nerve loses its myelin sheath (insulation) is when fats accumulate on top of it as plaque and steadily corrode it. B vitamins help move the fat through so it doesn't accumulate.

Biotin, choline, inositol, and thiamine are B vitamins that have all been found useful in treating diabetic neuropathy.

Researchers at the University of Athens discovered that regular, long-term use of the B vitamin biotin in diabetics was effective both for improvement in nerve conduction and relief of pain. Improvement was noted after 4 to 8 weeks of therapy.

Researchers at the University of Alabama saw significant improvement in nerve function in diabetics placed on a diet high in inositol. Included in the diet were high inositol foods, such as cantaloupe, peanuts, grapefruit, and whole grains. Robert Atkins, M.D., has reported his successful use of 2 to 6 grams per day for reversing diabetic neuropathy, and notes that physicians at St. James Hospital in Leeds, England have reported good results with even smaller dosages.

Thiamine has also been seen to be useful in treating diabetic neuropathy. Stanley Mirski, M.D., has reported that a large percentage of his diabetic patients who suffer from neuropathy have achieved improvements with daily thiamine supplementation in doses of 50 to 100 mg.

All of these B vitamins and more are included in Maximum Living's Vita Sprout formula and are derived from the kinds of foods diabetics should be eating. This food-based formula is far more effective than those that are derived from laboratory synthesized nutrients. Food and supplements that use food contain God's energy force. It's not just one nutrient that helps prevent disease, it's the combination of nutrients—as God intended—that delivers full life-sustaining force.

## ANTIOXIDANTS AND THE FAT CONNECTION

If you've ever smelled rotting meat, you know the effect fat, or cholesterol, has on the nervous system. The smell occurs as the meat oxidizes and turns rancid. When allowed to accumulate internally, fat essentially burns the nerves, or their protective covering, by releasing free radicals. Scientists call it Reactive Oxidative Stress (ROS). This is where antioxidants come in.

Alpha lipoic acid—a potent antioxidant—has long been used in Europe for the treatment of peripheral neuropathy in diabetics. A number of controlled clinical trials have shown its usefulness for reducing both the pain and numbness suffered by those with diabetic neuropathy. Its use for this condition is approved in Germany.

Another name for alpha lipoic acid is thioctic acid. In 1995, at a European conference, several speakers described the reversal of diabetic neuropathies using thioctic acid. They stated it was due to the nutrient's hypoglycemic and antioxidant effects. In German studies, researchers showed that thioctic acid regenerates nerve tissue and protects healthy neurons from the direct effect of high blood sugar.

In one research study, subjects with diabetic neuropathy were given a cocktail of antioxidants, including the mineral selenium, coenzyme Q10, beta-carotene, vitamin C, vitamin E, zinc, and vitamin B6. Sixty percent saw improvement.

Alpha-lipoic acid is included in Maximum Living's Antioxidant formula, as well as many of the nutrients you've been reading about in relation to diabetes and its symptomatic side effects.

Maximum Living also offers an excellent coenzyme Q10 formula.

Fight fat with essential fatty acids. Gamma linolenic acid (GLA) is an essential fatty acid found in borage oil, grape seed oil, black currant oil, and evening primrose oil that has been shown to be successful in reversing nerve damage in diabetics suffering from peripheral neuropathy. In a double-blind, placebo-controlled study using 480 milligrams of GLA daily, all of the diabetics given the fatty acid experienced gradual reversal of nerve damage and improvement in the symptoms related to the peripheral neuropathy, while those on placebo gradually worsened. It is thought that GLA may help to rebuild the myelin sheath around the nerves, thus restoring proper nerve conduction.

The best source of GLA is borage oil. Independent clinical tests show that borage oil contains up to 26 percent GLA. Compare this to evening primrose oil and black currant oil, which contain no more than 18 percent. Not only that, borage oil costs less because the borage seed is three times larger than black currant or evening primrose seeds. Finally, borage is more bioavailable. In other words, the body more readily accepts it. Two capsules of Maximum Living's Borage Oil contains 480 milligrams of GLA.

**MUST HAVE MINERALS**

Once again, the mineral magnesium is shown to help alleviate the affects of high blood sugar.

Magnesium is necessary for nerve conduction, and a deficiency is known to cause peripheral neuropathy symptoms. There have also been reports of chromium deficiency causing peripheral neuropathy. Selenium is a potent antioxidant mineral that helps alleviate the free radical burn of fatty deposits.

And, once again, I am reminding you that all the minerals must be taken in solution for optimal affect. MineralRich fits the bill especially well for nerve health, since it includes B12 as well as antioxidant minerals.

## Also in this Series

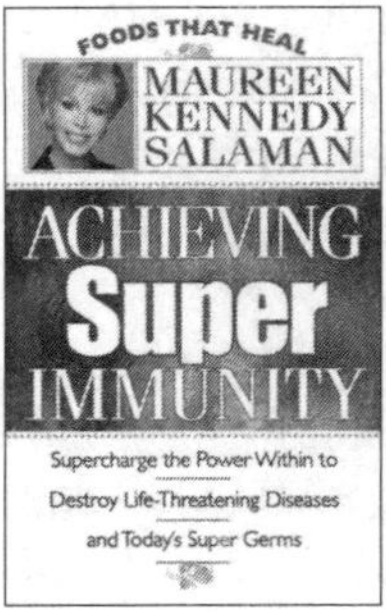


#610 / $7.95

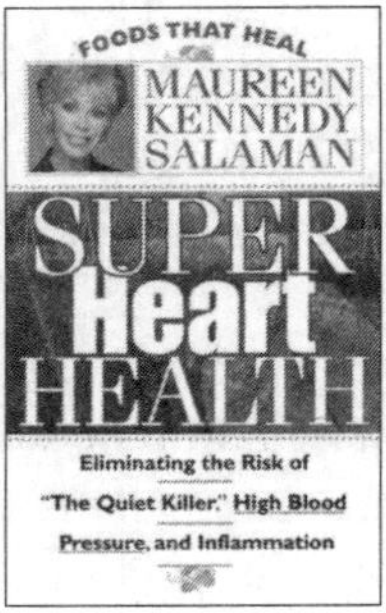


#625 / $7.95

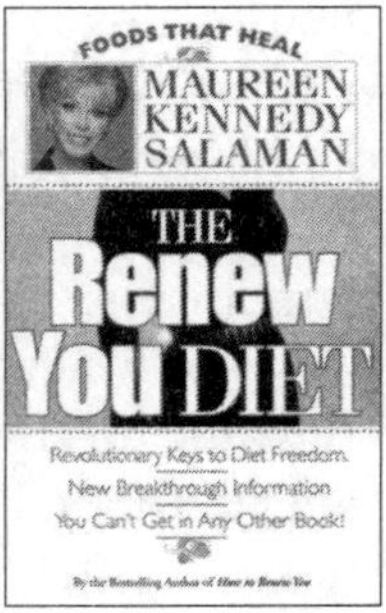


#620 / $7.95

OTHER BOOKS AVAILABLE

# INFORMATION PACKED BOOKS FOR HEALTHY LIVING

## *by Maureen Kennedy Salaman*

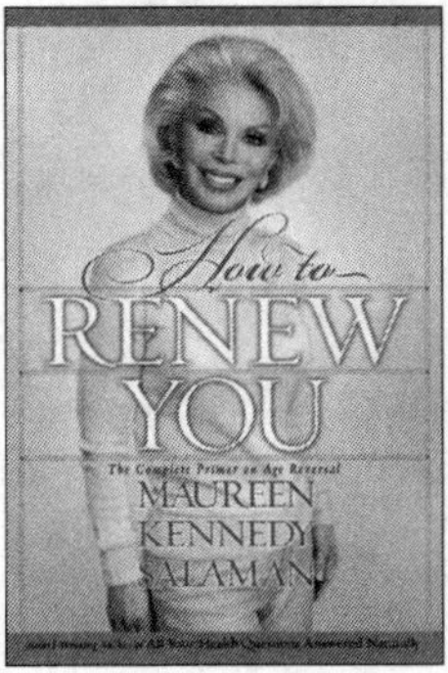


***How to Renew You: The Complete Primer on Age Reversal***
Do you wonder why some people sparkle with life and energy even at the age of 80 while others seem old at 50? Discover the secrets and success stories of staying perpetually youthful and glowing, no matter what your age, using these basic principles of renewal. Discover cutting edge research from medical scientists to us in your daily life. Rekindle, replenish, and rejuvenate you today!
**#570 / $19.95** paperback

***All Your Health Questions Answered Naturally***
The only nutritional encyclopedia and reference book you'll ever need. Others tell you what you already know, this book tells you what you need to know. Over 160 insightful chapters inform you of alternative and natural means not only to maintain and better your health but to help combat many ailments utilizing easy-to-follow methods.
**#550 / $29.95**

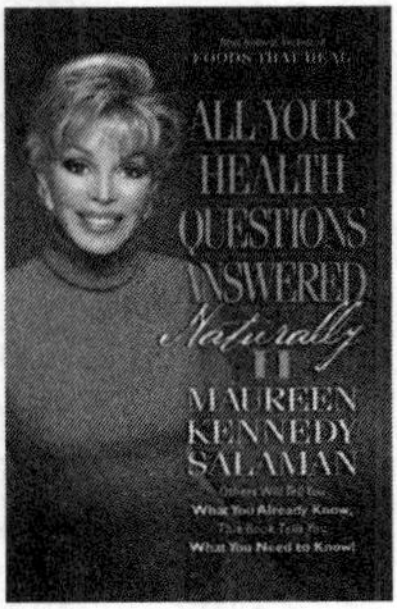


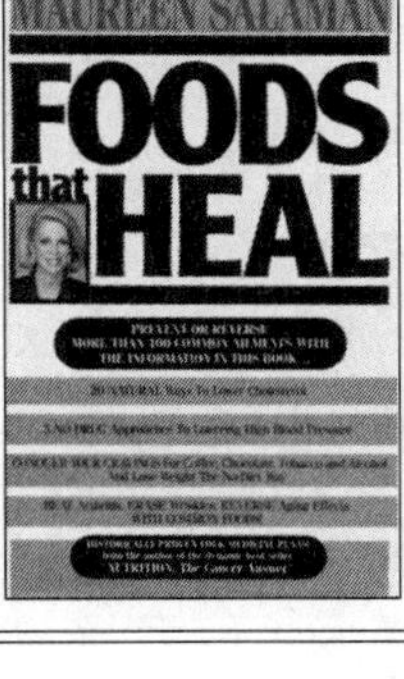


***Foods That Heal***
You can prevent and possibly reverse more than 100 common ailments by utilizing this thoroughly researched primer on divinely created natural foods. Learn how to combat arthritis, erase wrinkles, and reverse the effects of aging with common foods. This book details 5 non-drug based approaches to lowering high blood pressure and 20 natural ways to lower cholesterol. Discover natural means to conquer your cravings for coffee, chocolate, tobacco, and how to lose weight the "no-diet" way. **#510 / $19.95**